Diet for Tinnitus

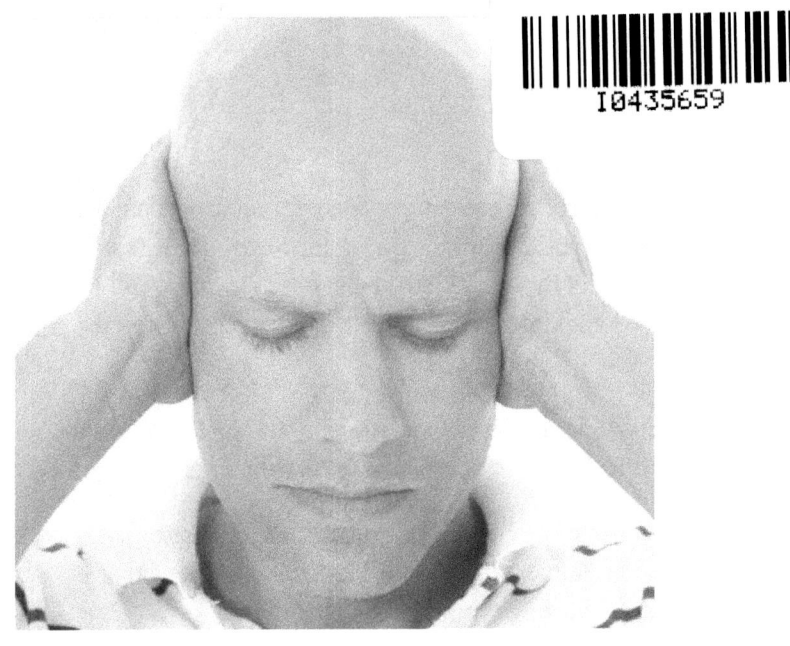

Health Learning Series

M. Usman

Mendon Cottage Books

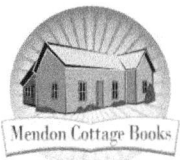

JD-Biz Publishing

All Images Licensed by Fotolia and 123RF.

Disclaimer

The information is this book is provided for informational purposes only. It is not intended to be used and medical advice or a substitute for proper medical treatment by a qualified health care provider. The information is believed to be accurate as presented based on research by the author.

The contents have not been evaluated by the U.S. Food and Drug Administration or any other Government or Health Organization and the contents in this book are not to be used to treat cure or prevent disease.

The author or publisher is not responsible for the use or safety of any diet, procedure, or treatment mentioned in this book. The author or publisher is not responsible for errors or omissions that may exist.

Warning

The Book is for informational purposes only and before taking on any diet, treatment or medical procedure, it is recommended to consult with your primary health care provider.

Our books are available at

1. Amazon.com
2. Barnes and Noble
3. Itunes
4. Kobo
5. Smashwords
6. Google Play Books

Table of Contents

Preface

Out of the five basic senses, one is hearing, without which undoubtedly we won't be living life to the fullest. The ears are incredible organs that allow a person to hear sounds; many times the organs are compared to radio dishes responsible for catching radio-waves and just like a radio-set, they too can sometimes become damaged.

One of the problems that can develop in the ears is tinnitus. Simply put, it is a condition in which the ear starts to listen to ringing, buzzing, and other meaningless noises. It is not dangerous nor a life-threatening condition, but with the passage of time the person will not get used to it but rather get annoyed by it. Moreover, untreated cases can cause damage to cognitive ability and increase restlessness in a person, turning his/her life into misery.

Tinnitus can be improved through treatment, both artificially and naturally. This book deals with the natural treatment of tinnitus, through proper diet, to be exact. Furthermore, you will get to know about the mechanism behind hearing, the types of tinnitus, how it gets diagnosed, and much more.

Stay tuned and keep reading.

Tinnitus

Chapter # 1: Hearing

Before we can go right into the mechanics of how our ears work in conjunction with other parts of the body (mostly the brain) to provide us with the ability to hear, a much simpler question needs to be answered.

What is sound?

The answer will be retorted in a simple manner; sound is a type of vibration that is produced in matter, i.e. solid, liquid and gas. Moreover, it can only pass through matter and cannot exist in space. It is heard by animals as soon as it reaches their ears. When an object vibrates in the air, it moves the air elements around it, which causes the subsequent air molecules to move. This is how eventually sound reaches you. This happens at an incredibly fast pace, i.e. about 450 meters per second!

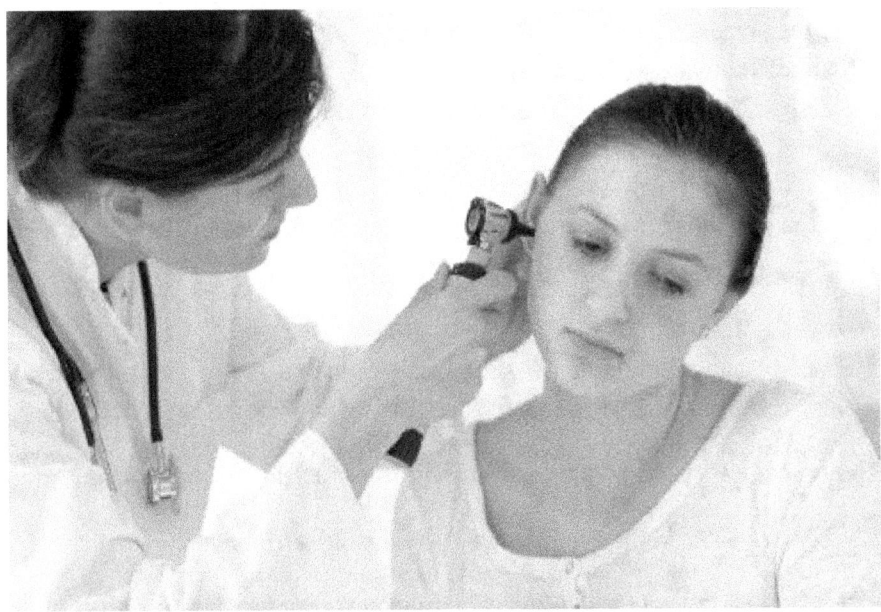

When a small stone is dropped in a static pond, ripples start to appear in an outward manner, originating from the point where the stone was initially dropped. Sound waves are of the invisible nature, but if somehow you were able to see them, they would be synonymous to the ripple-stone scenario stated earlier. As told earlier, sound waves cannot travel by themselves and need a medium to do so. This medium is usually the air present in our atmosphere; the atmosphere is made up of many gases in which sound can easily travel. In addition, sound can also travel through mediums like rocks (solid), or water (liquid).

Energy can never be created and at the same time never be destroyed, but what can be done is that it can change forms. The same principal applies here. For instance, do you know how human speech works? The larynx located in the throat has vocal cords and when air is allowed to pass through them, different frequencies are produced. When the vibrations are of low intensity, they have a deep resonating effect that is similar to the voices of men. In contrast, voices of higher intensity result in 'squeaky' and 'high-pitched' voices. The waves travel in all directions at a speed that is related to the air conditions, material density, etc.; normally the speed is close to 1200 km / hour.

Take the ubiquitous bell now. As soon as it is struck, the metal starts to vibrate both inwards and outwards. By moving towards one side, it replaces the air particles on that side. This leads to a chain reaction, with particles colliding into each other in turn, thus resulting in an action known as compression. Similarly, when the bell moves in the other direction it causes a decrease in the pressure and an increase in pressure on the other side resulting in a process known as rarefaction.

And this is how with the inclusion of these two processes, sound is produced. The different qualities of sound that are affected by the speed with which compressions occur include pitch, frequency, amplitude, etc.

Hence, our ears perform the following task in order to hear something:

i.   Take in the sound wave and transmit it to the hearing part.

ii.   Account for the fluctuations in air pressure.

iii.   Convert these air patterns into electric signals, which are then deciphered by the brain.

Chapter # 2: The Ear

You know how sound is produced and you know you receive it, but how does your ear give you such accurate perception of what it hears? What parts of the ear work together with the brain so that you can hear what you hear?

The ear is a mind-blowing organ. It consists of a multitude of thin string membranes which capture the slightest of vibrations. These membranes are located just inside the temporal bone separating the outer ear from the middle part; the membrane is widely referred to as ear drum. The ear drum might be very useful in the whole process, but at the same time, its high sensitivity makes it prone to injuries; it can get ripped apart from a foreign object or get damaged by high amplitude sounds.

The part of the ear one sees is nothing close to the real structure. The ear is structured into three tiers and is finely placed in the temporal bone. The eardrum captures sounds from the surroundings and transmits it to the inner part of the ear through an array of bones that act as amplifiers when the sound picked up is too weak or as padding when it's too loud. The outer part of the ear is pointed forward and it incorporates many curves. This arrangement has special meaning and helps the brain figure out the source of the sound. Sound coming from behind is reflected differently than that which comes sideways. When sound is picked up from a source lying laterally, your brain works out its horizontal position by processing data entered through both ears. If the source is present on the left side, it will reach the left ear more quickly than the right therefore it will be clearer in the left ear.

Naturally, a person is able to hear the sounds made in front of him/her more clearly than those generated at the their back. Mammals like dogs have flexible pinnae which allow them to focus on sounds in a much better way. However, this is not the case with humans and they are not that good at concentrating at sound sources. This does not mean that you can manually position your pinnae in another direction; humans can cup their ears which creates a greater surface area that ultimately helps the brain figure out the direction from which the sound originated in the first place.

The middle part of the brain is also uniquely structured in the sense that it is connected to our respiratory system! That's right; a canal connects the ear with the rest of the breathing network. The eardrum can rip off if there is a pressure difference between the ear's middle layer and outer layer therefore, the ear is engineered in a way that it preservers the pressure on both side. The eardrum being sensitive can easily be put to motion through the tiniest of vibrations. The ear drum is then connected to something known as tensor tympani muscle which pulls it towards the inside. The function of this muscle is to keep the eardrum material giving it uniformity no matter where the sound wave is struck. The eardrum is also known for its function of protecting the inner portion of the eyes. As soon as the brain figures out a very loud noise incoming, it pulls in the eardrum to make it as stiff as possible so that minimum sound will enter the ear.

Now is the inner tier, which is considered one of the most complicated parts of the body. The section is filled with a network of bones that form a shape similar to a snail's shell. This inner part serves two functions: it converts sound and it acts as a gyroscope. The latter part means, that a sense of balance is given to the body by this part of the ear. This part of the ear can easily get infected and thus needs great care and protection.

Next, you'll see how simply tinnitus strikes and can turn into a condition that can turn your life into psychological misery.

Chapter # 3: Enter Tinnitus

Tinnitus is one of the first signs of ear problems in elderly people. Sometimes it's a side effect of a disease, while sometimes of medications. Over 200 drugs have been categorized to contain compounds that cause tinnitus. The condition itself is commonly described as a buzzing, hissing, roaring, or a ringing sound in the ear. It may be of variable loudness and pitch and may be present in only one ear. In the past year alone over 22 million adults in America suffered from tinnitus for a period of more than 3 months; this accounts for 10 percent of the population in the US.

People who work in noisy and loud places like construction sites, heavy mechanical factories, or auditoriums can often develop tinnitus with the passage of time due to exposure to excessive noises. This damages the sensory cells located in the inner ear that result in the disruption of sound transmitted to the brain. The condition is known as **Noise-induced hearing loss**. Soldiers exposed to blasts and firing drills can develop tinnitus quite easily as the shockwave produced in battlefield can easily damage cells in the brain that help receive sound. It is for this reason that this type of tinnitus is very common in war veterans.

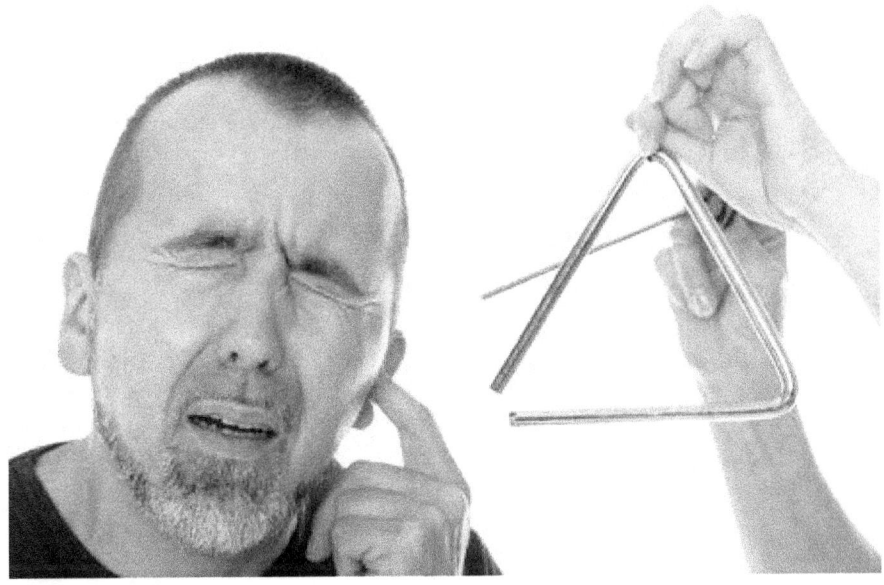

Another type of tinnitus is **pulsatile tinnitus,** which is the formation of a rhythmic pulsating sound in the ear; synchronized with one's heartbeat. A doctor is able to check this type of tinnitus by placing a stethoscope pressed against a person's neck. He/she examines the blood flow to the brain, as this is one of the most common causes of this type of tinnitus. Furthermore, pulsatile tinnitus may also be caused due to brain diseases.

Even though tinnitus is heard in our ears, it really starts off in the brain or as the scientists call it, the neural network. Scientists believe that the brain actually creates an illusion that a sound is present, when it actually isn't, leading to tinnitus. Tinnitus can also be caused due to the brain's neural network trying to make up for the loss of cells that receive sound by making parts of the ear more sensitive; this results in an oversensitive ear that ultimately leads to tinnitus. It may also be a case of out of balance neural circuits when the inner ear has been damaged; a part of the brain that processes sound.

Tinnitus may be caused by a number of diseases, ailments, and medications. These are explained in the forthcoming chapter.

Chapter # 4: Causes of Tinnitus

There are a number of conditions that can cause or actually worsen the effects of tinnitus. Most of the times the exact condition is never found, but still scientists have been able to round up some of the most common causes of tinnitus. Most of the times, tinnitus is caused by:

- **Exposure to noise** – Loud noises like those of chain saws, bomb-explosions, etc. can cause noise-related hearing loss. Media devices like iPods, mp3 players, if heard for a great length of time, can result in hearing loss. This type of tinnitus is caused by exposure to sounds for a temporary period of time; however, if the ear has to deal with these sounds on a regular basis, they can cause permanent damage.

- **Age-related hearing loss** – Similar to many other parts of body, with the passage of time, hearing also worsens. This happens close to the age of 60, and is known as presbycusis.

- **Ear bone changes** – In the middle part of your ear, your bones can become stiff which can result in difficulties in hearing. This problem usually runs within the families.

- **Earwax blockage** – Earwax is known to protect the ear canal by slowing the growth of bacteria and trapping dirt in it. When too much earwax builds up, it can cause hearing loss as it can no longer be washed off naturally, leading to tinnitus.

- **Meniere's disease** – This is an inner ear disorder which causes abnormal ear fluid pressure.

- **TMJ disorder** – The temporomandibular joint which meets up with lower jawbone at your neck can sometimes be damaged leading to tinnitus.

- **Head or Neck injuries** – Trauma to the neck or ear can result in tinnitus.

- **Acoustic neuroma** – This is a benign form of tumor which is formed on the cranial nerve, present throughout the passageway from the brain to the ear. The nerve controls hearing and balance, and the tumor can disrupt its normal functions leading to tinnitus.

- **Atherosclerosis** – Cholesterol can buildup in any blood vessel in the body; sometimes it buildups in the middle ear that results in the loss of the ear's elasticity. This causes the blood flow to apply more shear force than it normally does, resulting in damage to the ear. This type of tinnitus generally occurs in both ears.

- **High blood pressure** – Hypertension or high blood pressure can magnify the effects of tinnitus and make it more noticeable.

- **Turbulence in blood pressure** – Tinnitus can also be caused due to narrowing of the blood vessel that provides blood to the ears.

- **Malfunctioning capillaries** – A condition known as AVM or arteriovenous malformation can cause weird connections between different veins in the body that results in tinnitus; this usually occurs in one ear.

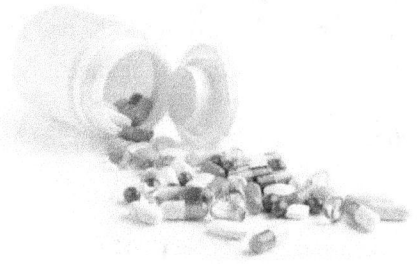

Other than ailments and conditions, medications are also known to cause tinnitus; the higher the dose of a particular medicine, the worse the case becomes. Medications known to induce tinnitus include:

- **Cancer medications** – like vincristine and mechlorethamine.

- **Antibiotics** – like neomycin, Vancomycin, polymyxin B and erythromycin.

- **Diuretics** – like ethacrynic acid, bumetanide, or furosemide.

- **Quinine medications** – like those for malaria.

- **Anti-depressants**.

- **Aspirin** – if abused or near the maximum limit. (12 or more per day).

A Healthy Diet

Tinnitus might not be much of a problem initially, but soon it will start giving you episodes of depression, headaches, and annoyance that will make it unbearable. Many techniques have been put forward for the treatment of tinnitus, but one has greatly stood out: lifestyle. By changing your lifestyle, you can literally see huge differences in your health and the main factor that describes a person's lifestyle is his/her diet. A healthy diet filled with vitamins, minerals and all the beneficial nutrients can greatly decrease the risk of tinnitus and help cure it if it's already there.

From fruits to vegetables, grains to fats, this chapter will explain about all the right things that should be a part of your diet in order to make a recovery back to normalcy.

Chapter # 1: Fruits & Vegetables

In almost all of the developing and developed countries, more and more people are inclined towards pre-cooked snacks, rather than fruits and vegetables. Most people have completely ignored vegetables to a level that they eat it only in the form of onions, lettuce, and tomatoes in burgers. This attitude needs to be changed and all your snacks must contain abundant green vegetables like spinach, broccoli, and sprouts. Similarly, tinnitus sufferers must use mushrooms, eggplants, and sweet potatoes in their diet as well. The secret of this food group lies in the vitamins they contain and in this case they are rich with vitamin A which is known for its ability to restore the scratched surface of the eardrums. Moreover, vitamin E is of considerable importance in treating tinnitus.

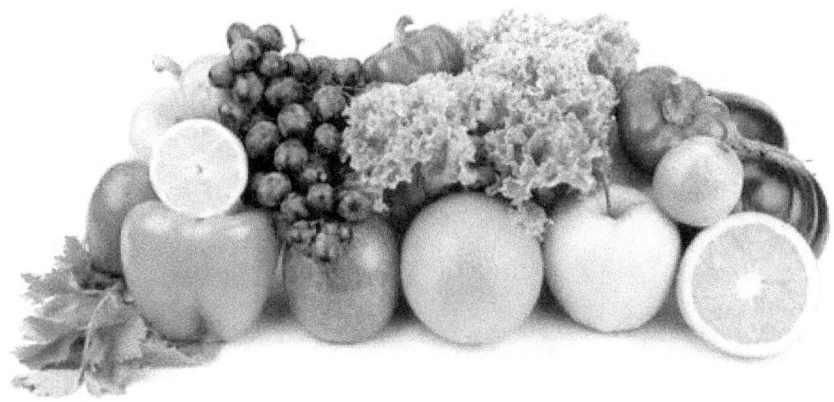

Along with vegetables, fruits can deliciously help you deal with tinnitus. Regardless of how you consume fruits, they will increase your oxygen levels and blood flow that are required for a healthy inner ear. They will boost your body health through B-vitamins and no preparation is required for these fruits, just eat them raw.

Fruits and vegetables rich in vitamin A, B and K include:

Sweet potato	Romaine Lettuce

Carrots	Tropical Fruit
Kale	Red peppers
Spinach	Dried apricots
Broccoli	Grapefruit juice
Pineapple	Orange

Chapter # 2: Grains, Legumes, Herbs & Fats

Grains are necessary for a proper, balanced diet. They are known to improve brain functions linked to processing our ears and if included in the diet, they can provide the body with ample amounts of fibers, proteins, vitamin B, and omega fats. Moreover they are great for one's heart and the circulatory system, which ultimately ensures proper blood circulation in all parts of the body. A well-fueled brain will, in essence, be sharper and thus more focused, annoying any buzzing sounds created by tinnitus. Don't ever ignore whole grains, if you wish to conquer tinnitus, as they are absolutely essential to maintain proper bodily functions. The following grains should be included in your diet for providing you with the essential nutrients for a healthy ear:

i. Oatmeal,

ii. Millet,

iii. Rye,

iv. Quinoa,

v. Brown rice

Legumes are one of the most commonly eaten materials day to day for most people. No matter how much you try, in one way or another you will eventually consume legumes. While many legumes are beneficial for the body, for tinnitus sufferers, two stand out: peas and beans. There are hundreds of variations of peas and beans, but over here only the ones that help a person with hearing are discussed. The beans and peas can be divided further into 2 categories with respect to the vitamins they contain:

Vitamin B	Vitamin C
Adzuki beans	Split peas
Black beans	Soy beans
Black eye peas	Navy beans

Lima beans	Kidney beans
Mung beans	Chick peas
Pigeon peas	Garbanzo beans
White beans	Fava beans

Apart from containing vitamins the beans are also rich in minerals like phosphorous, potassium, magnesium, and calcium. They are perfect as a side dish and more importantly very affordable.

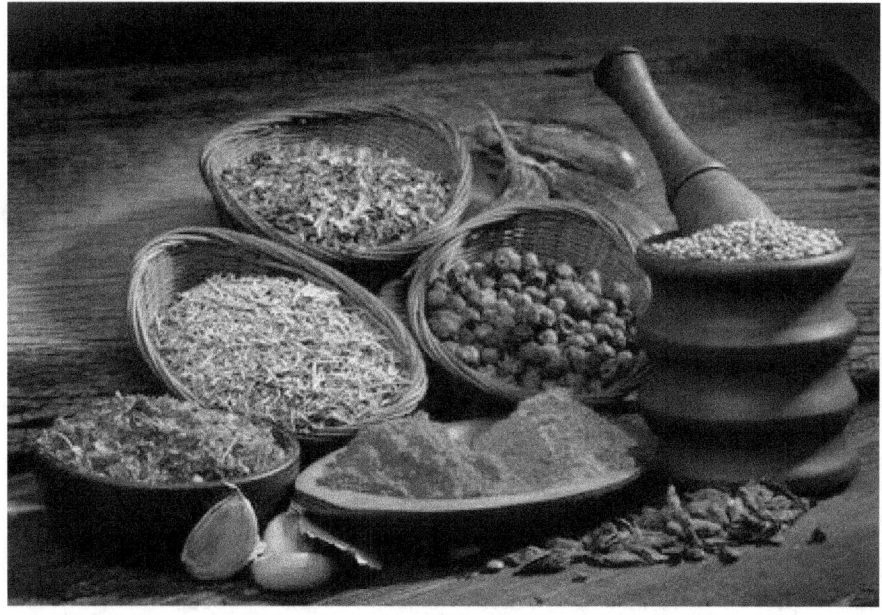

Seasoning one's food is always considered that part of cooking that has no health benefit. This is wrong, as every herb and spice you use as a garnish has its potential implications on your health. The seasonings not only make the food tastier but also help in the treatment of tinnitus. The herbs and spices are an affordable treatment for tinnitus and they can easily be integrated in one's diet by sprinkling over every food. The following are 5 spices very beneficial to sufferers of tinnitus:

- Cinnamon

- Black pepper

- Nutmeg

- Paprika

- Turmeric

Still, it's important to make sure that you are not allergic to any one of these spices.

Also a very powerful spice that can be used as a great treatment for tinnitus is Wolfberry. It is a red berry available in China that is used in different cereals and grains to fight against tinnitus. The berries are really packed with antioxidants that are beneficial for the ear, but it cannot be used by diabetics and people with high blood pressure.

Now are the fats. The popular belief says that fats are bad for the health and can never be associated with a healthy lifestyle. This is not entirely correct as numerous fats that a person consumes in his day to day life are beneficial to his/her body. There are four types of fat out of which two are considered healthy. The following is a table that illustrates the difference between the two:

Healthy Fats		Unhealthy Fats	
Monounsaturated Fats	Poly-saturated Fats	Trans fats	Saturated fats
Avocados	Fatty fish	Butter	Quick foods
Olives	Tofu	Whipped cream	Margarine
Sunflower seeds	Soymilk	Lard	Fast food
Peanut butter	Walnuts	Palm oil	Deep fried meat
Peanuts	Seafood	Ice cream	Candy bards

Nuts	Flaxseeds	Coconut oil	Industrial dough

Based on this table, it would become quite easy for you to make a comprehensive meal plan as to which fat you'll use each day.

Chapter # 3: Dairy, Meats & Seafood

A breakfast is not complete without eggs and milk, period. Most people can't even live with the idea of not having these two food items at their table in the morning, and with these people lies the secret of staying healthy. Eggs and milk contain essential proteins and vitamins that can help cure tinnitus; egg whites are perfect for this condition as they contain 8 essential acids. Thus tinnitus sufferers must have dairy in their regular diet and if there's a problem like lactose intolerance, shift to alternatives like soy milk. Furthermore, tinnitus sufferers should try to avoid cow's milk and drink goat or sheep milk as it is more beneficial to the body. Compared to goat's milk, cow milk contains less b vitamins, minerals that are essential for tinnitus to heal.

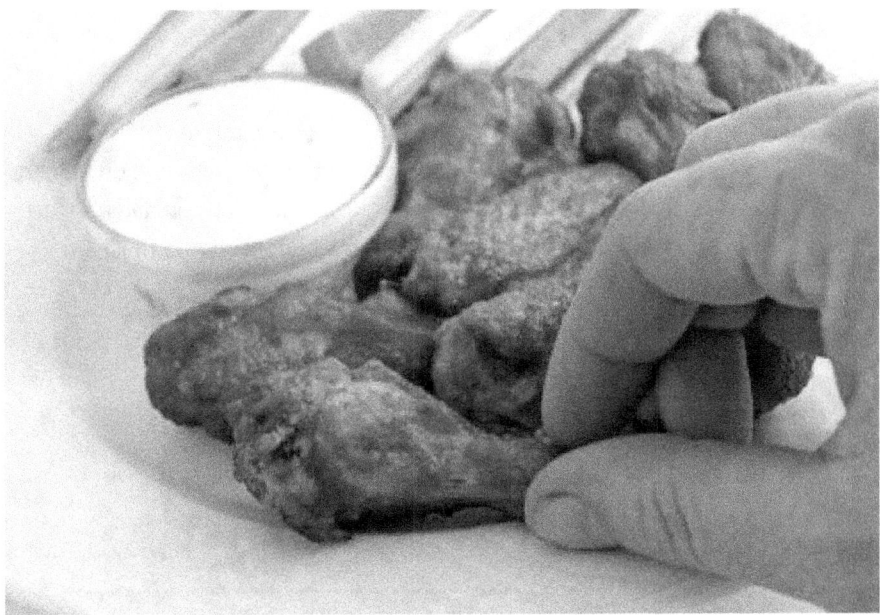

Lean meats aren't that much healthier when compared to the rest of the food groups, yet still they are considered one of the greatest sources of iron. The iron is an essential mineral, without which a person can suffer from hemorrhages. This condition can then become a cause of tinnitus and other ear conditions. The iron deficiency can be filled with the consumption of myoglobin which is a protein found in the muscles of mammals as well as birds. Chicken meat can be introduced in one's diet to fix this problem, but still chicken meat contains a very low percentage compared to beef meat which contains as high as 3%. That's not all and meats are also known to contain, vitamin D, phosphorous, zinc and other minerals that can alleviate hearing problems related to tinnitus.

Fish and seafood are also very beneficial for tinnitus' sufferers and can become an integral part of your diet. Firstly, there are fish that come from lakes and rivers known as fresh water fish. These include fish like salmon, tarpon, catfish, carp, etc. Then, a wider variety of fish found in oceans:

- Fish like tuna, cod and shark,

- Mollusks like sea nails, clams and squids,

- Crustaceans like shrimps, lobsters and crabs,

- Aquatic plants like seaweed

Both white and oily fish will provide the body with abundant levels of proteins, selenium, and phosphorous that will help in keeping the cholesterol down. This in turn will lead to better blood flow in the body including parts of the brain and ear that will ultimately lead to a better hearing ability.

Chapter # 4: Others

Last, but definitely not least, you should consume as much tea as possible. It has been used since ancient times to cure ailments and deal with diseases. There are three types of teas that should be consumed by tinnitus sufferers. These include:

i. Green tea:

Being one of the most respected types of tea, green tea is consumed by both Western and Eastern civilizations. Green tea is known to positively affect blood circulation and prevent arterial diseases that can cause tinnitus.

ii. Fenugreek tea:

This particular tea is one of the most widely used natural remedies in the fight against tinnitus. At first it was only popular in Asia, but now its fame has spread across the world. The remedy won't heal you of tinnitus completely but will sure help you deal with it in a better way.

iii. Ginkgo Biloba tea:

This is an ancient Chinese plant whose antioxidant affects are famous for curing many diseases; it has proven especially good for circulation of blood in the brain and is one of the main reasons used to protect the body from tinnitus.

Eating all the right foods is not the answer; you should also try your best to leave behind all the things that are causing tinnitus in the first place. These include items like:

- Coffee,

- Cigarettes,

- Salt,

- Unwanted medications,

- Alcohol,

- Illicit drugs.

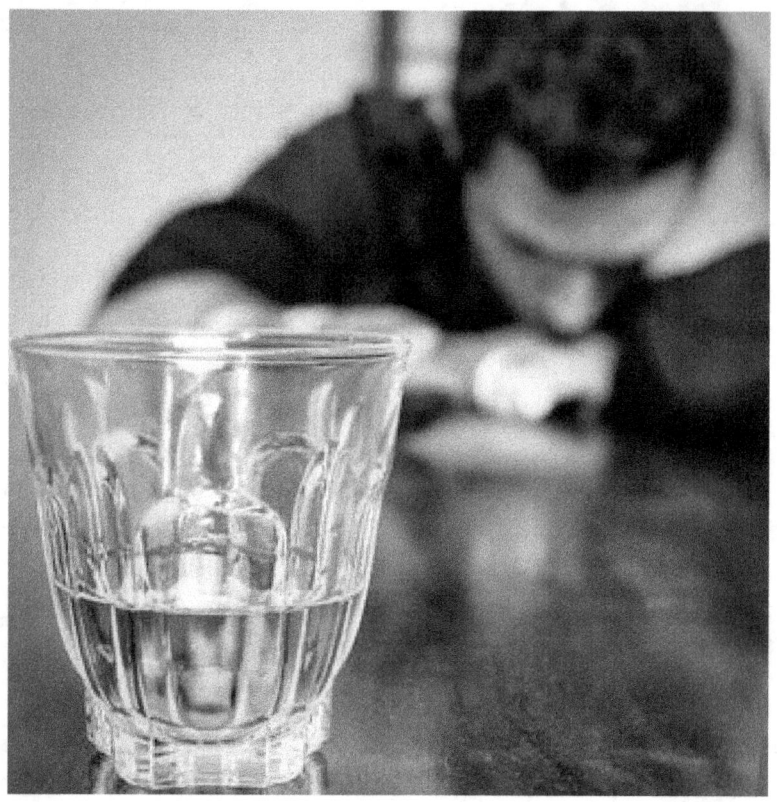

Recipes

Chapter # 1: Carrot & Lentil Soup

Makes: 4 servings

Prep time: 10 minutes

Cooking time: 15 minutes

Ingredients:

- 2 teaspoon cumin seeds,

- 2 tablespoon olive oil,

- A pinch of chili flakes

- 140 grams red lentils,

- 600 grams carrots

- 1 vegetable stock

- 125 ml milk

- Plain yogurt

Directions:

Firstly, heat a large saucepan and fry the cumin seeds along with the chili flakes for one minute or until they begin to show signs of motion in and around the pan. Scoop out half of the seeds using a spoon and set them aside. Add carrots, lentils, stock, milk, and oil to the pan, bringing it to a boil after that. Let it simmer for 15 minutes or until the lentils are swollen. Use a food processor or a stick blender to whizz the soup. Season it with a dollop of yogurt or sprinkle a few spices over it. Serve with naan.

Chapter # 2: Coriander & Lamb Curry

Makes: 4 servings

Prep time: 15 minutes

Cooking time: 60 minutes

Ingredients:

- 750 grams lamb in 3 cm cubes,

- 1 ½ teaspoon turmeric,

- 280 grams Greek yogurt,

- 2 cloves crushed garlic,

- 2 large chopped onions,

- 2 ½ tablespoons vegetable oil,

- ½ teaspoon chili powder,

- 4 large tomatoes,

- 40 grams roasted cashews,

- 2 ½ teaspoon ground coriander,

- 100 grams *paneer*,

- ½ cup coriander

Directions:

First, make the lamb tikka by combining the yogurt, lamb, ½ of the garlic, and a teaspoon of turmeric in a medium sized bowl. Cover and place in the refrigerator for 30 minutes. Next, heat a tablespoon of oil in a large frying pan over medium heat and scrape off any leftover marinade from the lamb, cooking in 2 batches for 3 minutes or until desired stage reached. To make the curry, heat the remaining oil in a saucepan, and add the remaining garlic, stirring for 30 seconds or until the garlic becomes fragrant. Add in the onions and cook for 30 minutes this time, until the onions are dark golden in color. Next, add the salt, chili, turmeric and coriander, cooking for 1 minute; the tomatoes and water go in next followed by the lamb to the pan. Let it simmer for 15 minutes.

To give the curry more enrichment, process the paneer, water, and cashews in a food processor to make a paste. Add the coriander leaves and stir this paste, cooking for 5 more minutes. Serve this curry with bread.

Chapter # 3: Pasta alongside Lentil Sauce

Makes: 4 servings

Prep time: 10 minutes

Cooking time: 25 minutes

Ingredients:

- 2 tablespoons olive oil,

- 1 carrot, chopped

- 1 onion, chopped

- 2 sticks of celery,

- 2 garlic cloves,

- 2 teaspoons cumin,

- 1 tablespoon tomato paste,

- 410 grams brown lentils,

- 800 grams canner tomatoes,

- 100 grams feta,

- 300 grams spaghetti,

Directions:

First, heat the olive oil in a sauce pan over medium heat. Next, add in the carrot, onion, and celery, cooking for 5 minutes over low heat. Add the cumin, garlic, tomatoes, and paste followed by ½ cup of water. Bring the water to a boil and season with salt. Turn the heat down and let it simmer for 10 minutes before adding the lentils and cooking once again for 5 minutes. In the meantime, cook the spaghetti according to the packet instructions. Divide the spaghetti in serving bowls and serve with feta.

Chapter # 4: Moroccan Chickpea Soup

Makes: 4 servings

Prep time: 5 minutes

Cooking time: 20 minutes

Ingredients:

- 1 tablespoon olive oil,

- 2 celery sticks,

- 1 medium onion,

- 2 teaspoon ground cumin,

- 400 grams chopped tomatoes,

- 600 ml vegetable stock,

- 100 grams broad beans,

- Zest,

- Lemon juice

- Coriander and parsley, a handful

Directions:

Heat the oil in a medium sized saucepan and fry the celery and onions in it for 10 minutes, or until it is softened. Add in the cumin, and let it fry for 1 more minute. Turn up the heat and toss in the tomatoes, chickpeas, and stock. Let it simmer for 8 minutes before adding the lemon juice and broad beans; cook for 2 more minutes. Season with salt and pepper as desired and top it with lemon zests.

Chapter # 5: South-Western Salad

Makes: 2 servings

Prep time: 20 minutes

Cooking time: 10 minutes

Ingredients:

- 2 sweet corn,

- 1 avocado,

- 400 grams black beans,

- 200 grams halved cherry tomatoes,

- 100 grams crumbled feta cheese,

- 4 chopped spring onions,

- Lime wedges

For the dressing:

- 1 tablespoon chipotle Tabasco sauce,

- 1 teaspoon ground cumin,

- 1 tablespoon sherry vinegar,

- 2 tablespoon olive oil,

- Juice and zest

Directions:

Boil the corn in salted water for approximately 10 minutes; rinse in cold water and cut the kernels. Add the beans in a bowl with the cooked avocado, corn, spring onions, and tomatoes. Mix the ingredients for dressings and pour it over the salad. Toss it together and sprinkle the feta cheese over it; serve with the lime wedges.

Conclusion

Tinnitus is an ear disorder that is not life threatening, but has a devastating effect on a person's day to day life. It strikes as a hissing, buzzing sound in one's ear that soon starts to take the life out of him/her. It disturbs the person's sleep patterns, work life, and also personal life. Many treatments have come forward to help patients with tinnitus but only one, natural treatment has stood out: following a healthy diet. Correcting one's diet is the only way to truly prevent and alleviate the effects of tinnitus. The details of the diet have been given in the book which should act as a guideline for you whenever, you have an ambiguity about tinnitus or the food groups allowed by its diet. In the end, you have to stay motivated to truly make a difference.

Best of luck!

References

http://nl.123rf.com/photo_11545080_aantrekkelijke-man-houdt-zijn-oren-dicht-alle-op-een-witte-achtergrond.html?term=tinnitus

http://nl.123rf.com/photo_14904087_kno-arts-kijkt-in-het-oor-van-de-patia-nt-met-een-instrument.html?term=ear

http://nl.123rf.com/photo_31435518_een-driehoekje-naast-het-hoofd-van-een-man-in-doodsangst.html?term=tinnitus

http://fotolia.com/id/45417819

http://fotolia.com/id/45901427

http://fotolia.com/id/47170066

http://fotolia.com/id/11347590

http://fotolia.com/id/51912489

Author Bio

Muhammad Usman is a distinguished medical graduate of Allama Iqbal medical college (AIMC). He is a professional writer who has been in the field for more than 4 years. During this time he has produced 10,000+ articles, blogs, and eBooks on various niches related to diseases, health, fitness, nutrition, and well-being. He is a regular contributor to several journals related to medicine and surgery. He is the editor of several journals and newspapers.

Check out some of the other JD-Biz Publishing books

Gardening Series on Amazon

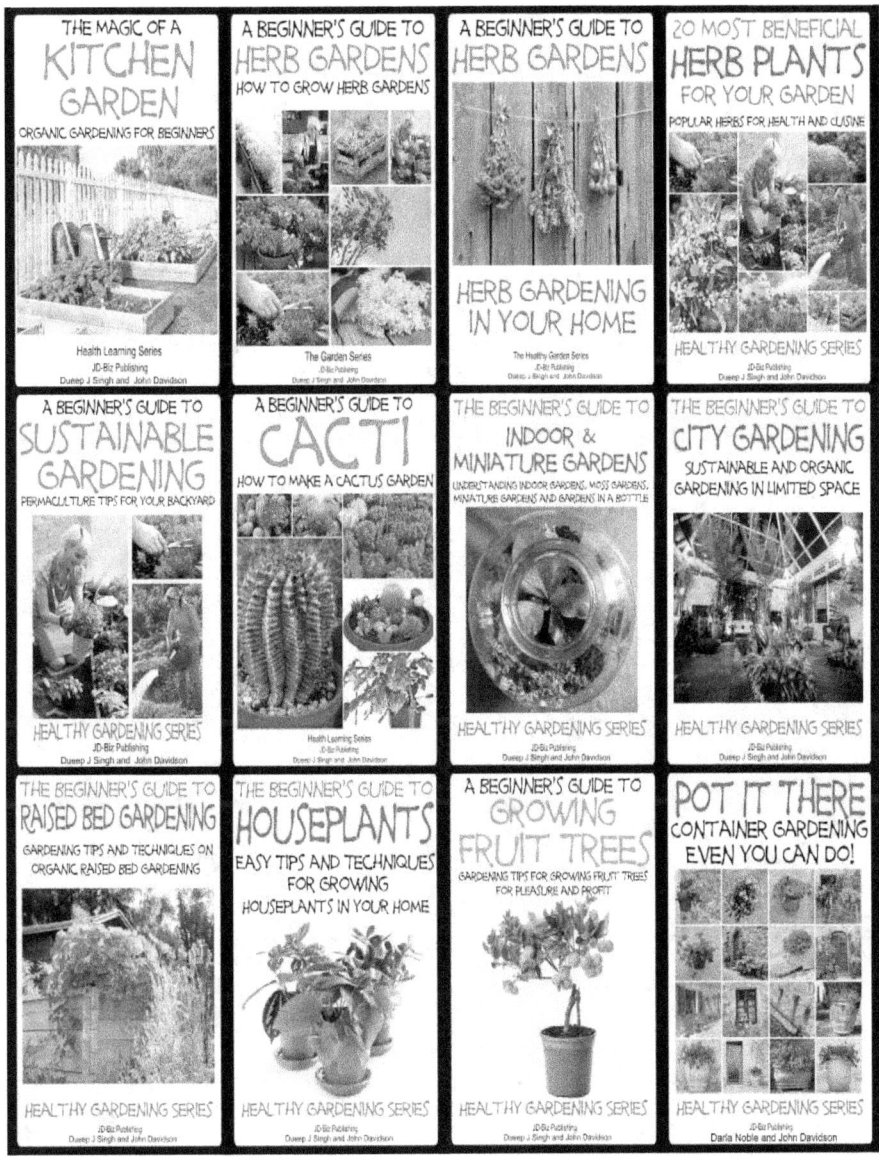

Health Learning Series

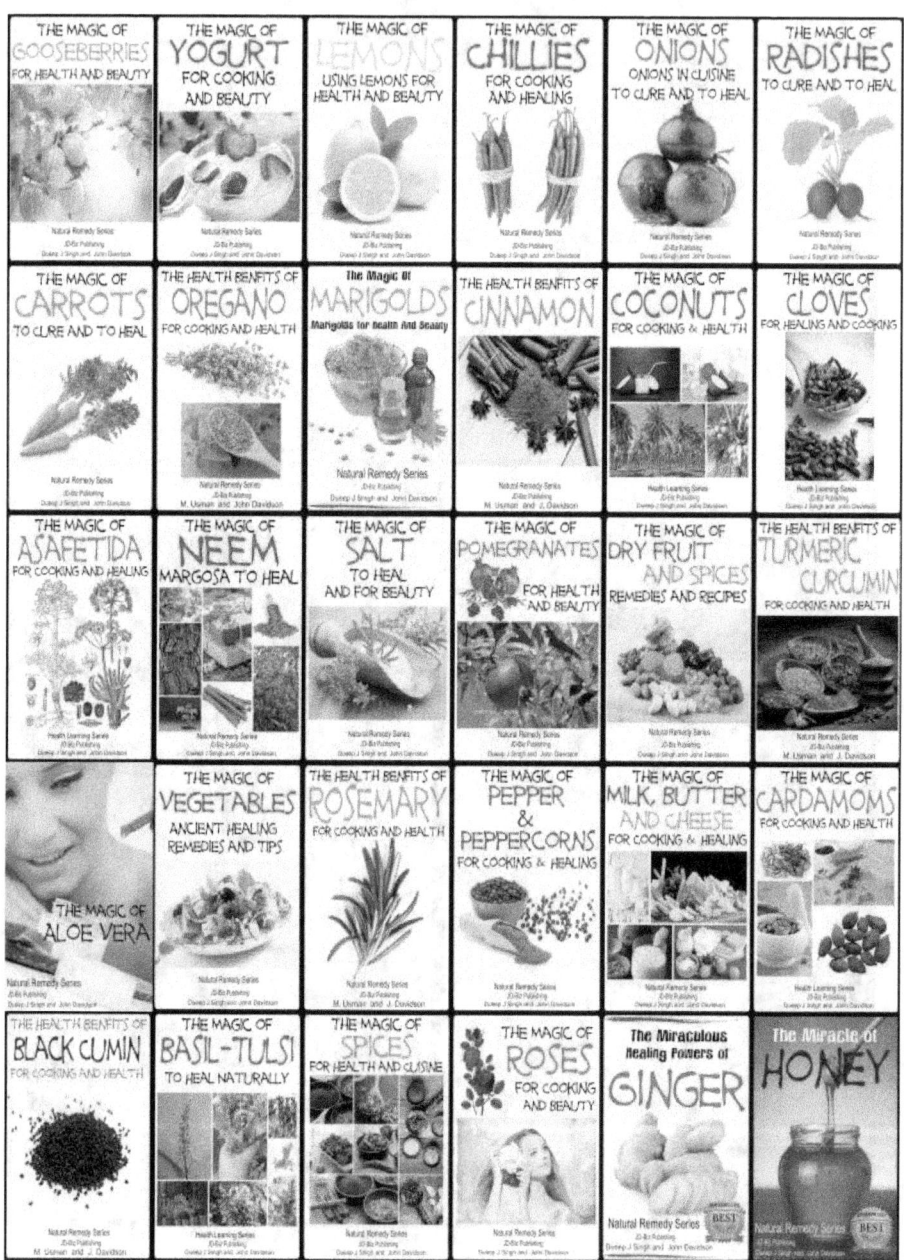

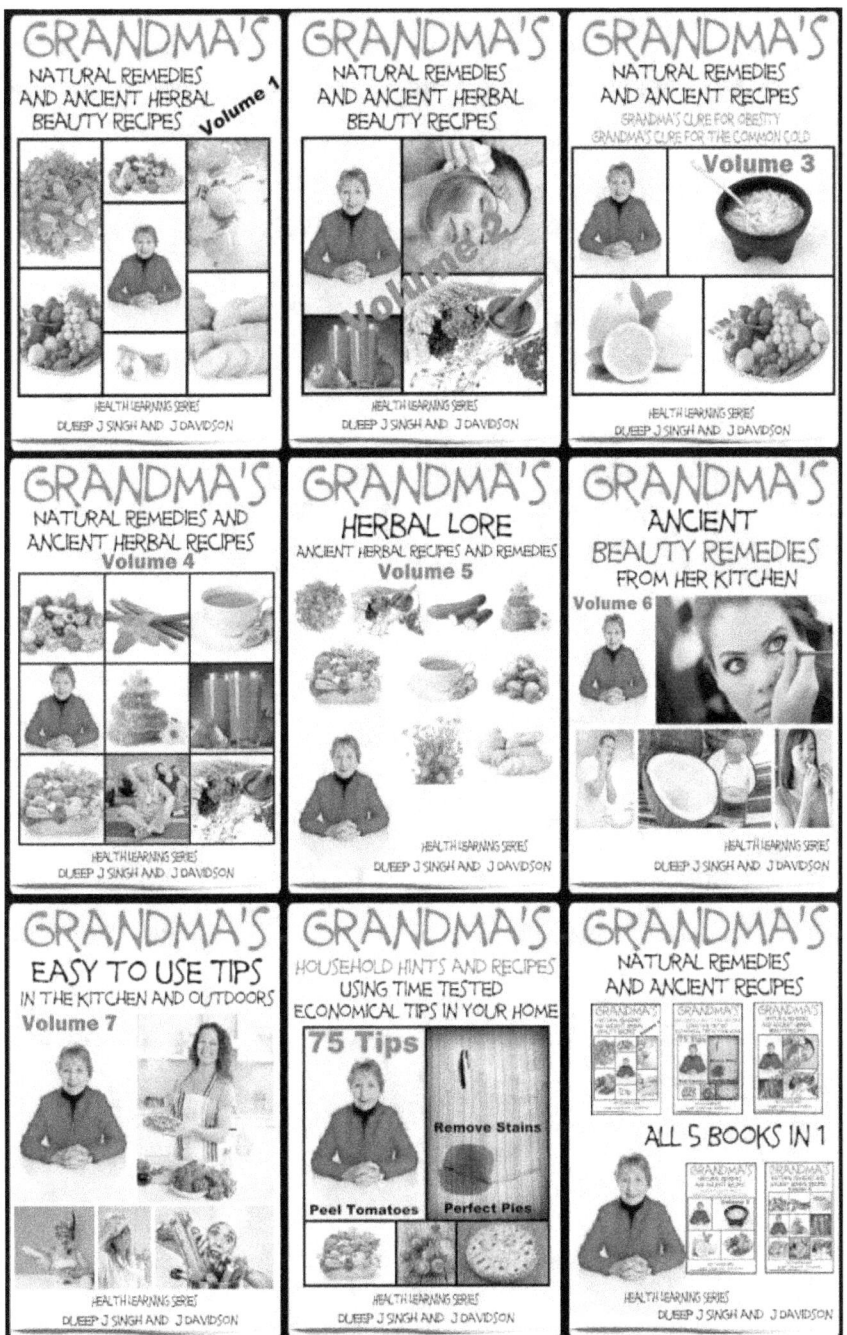

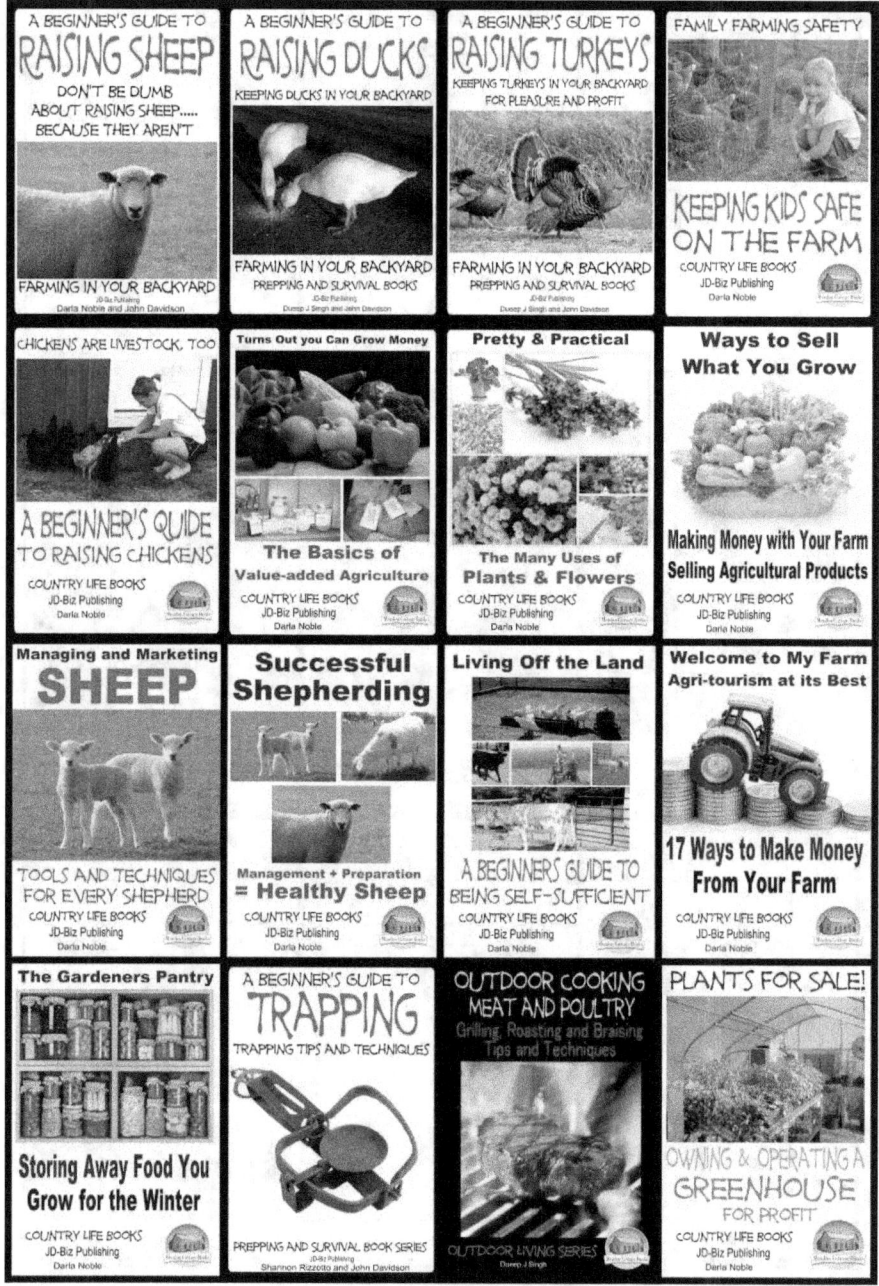

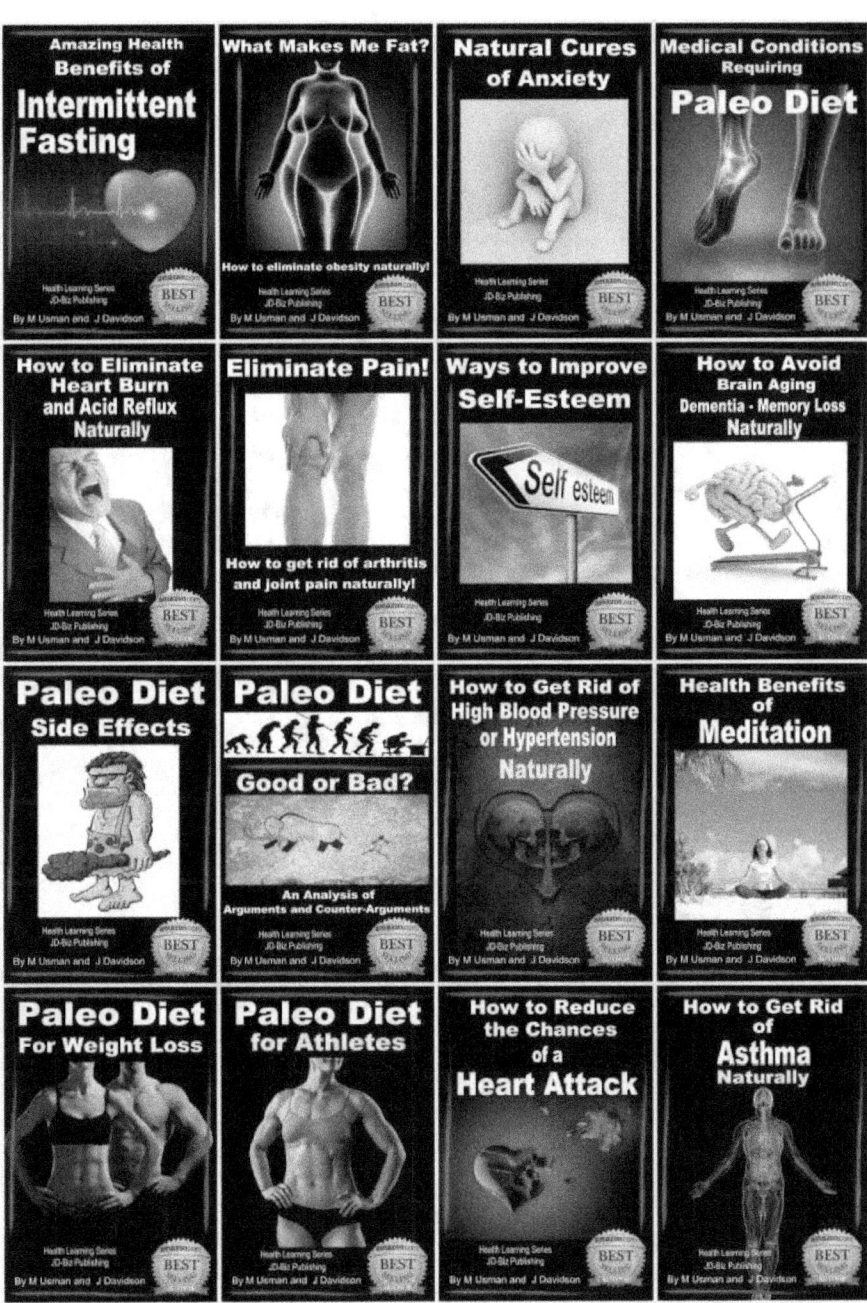

Amazing Animal Book Series

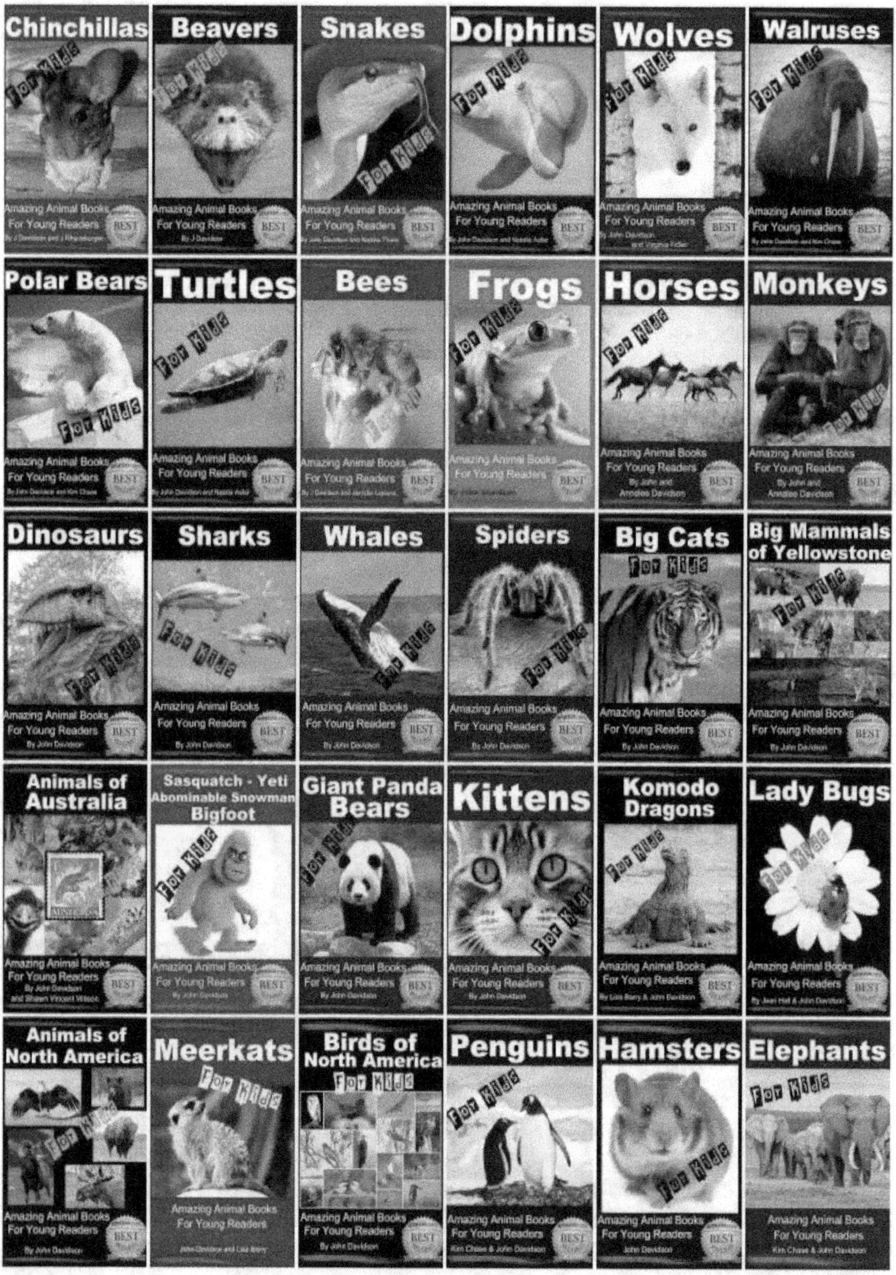

Learn To Draw Series

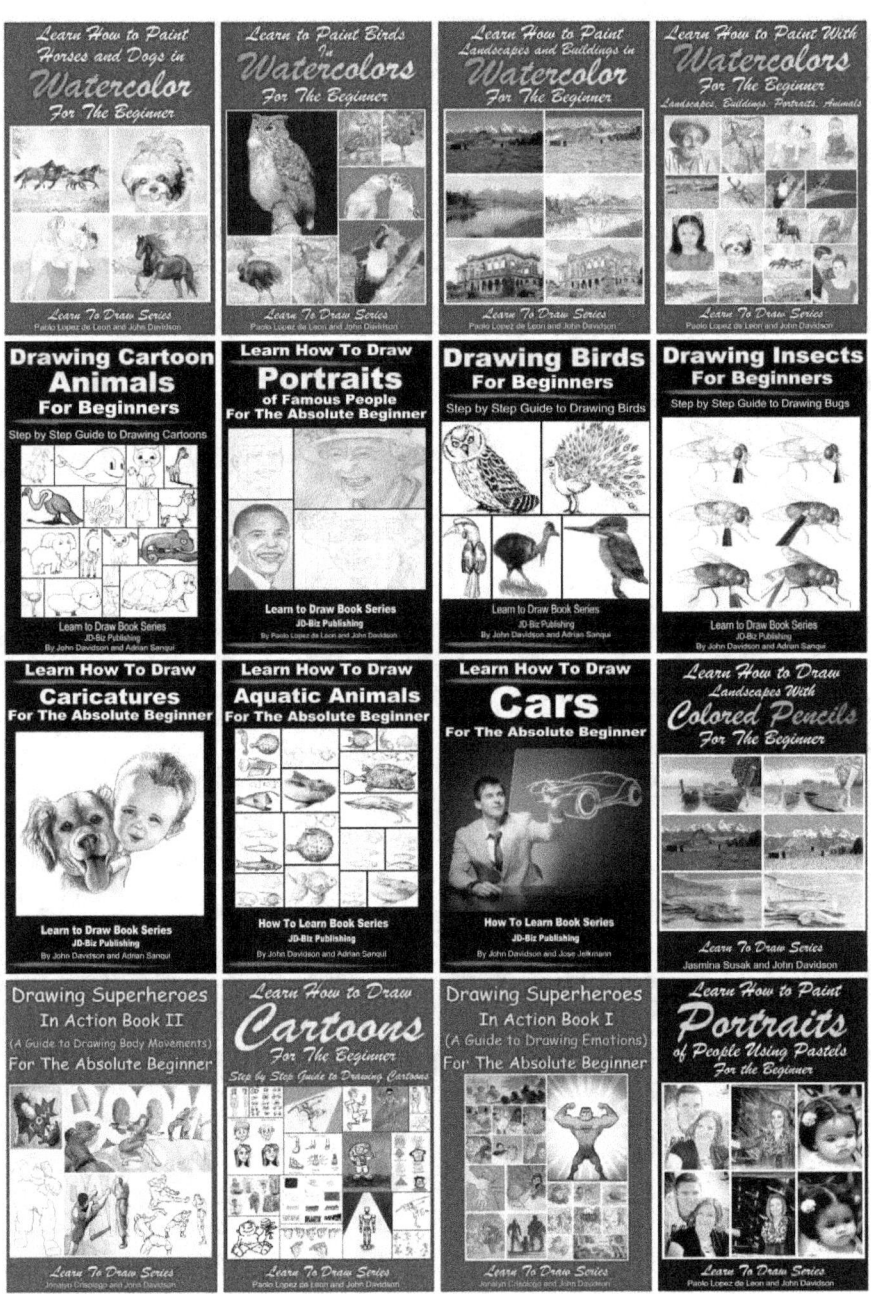

How to Build and Plan Books

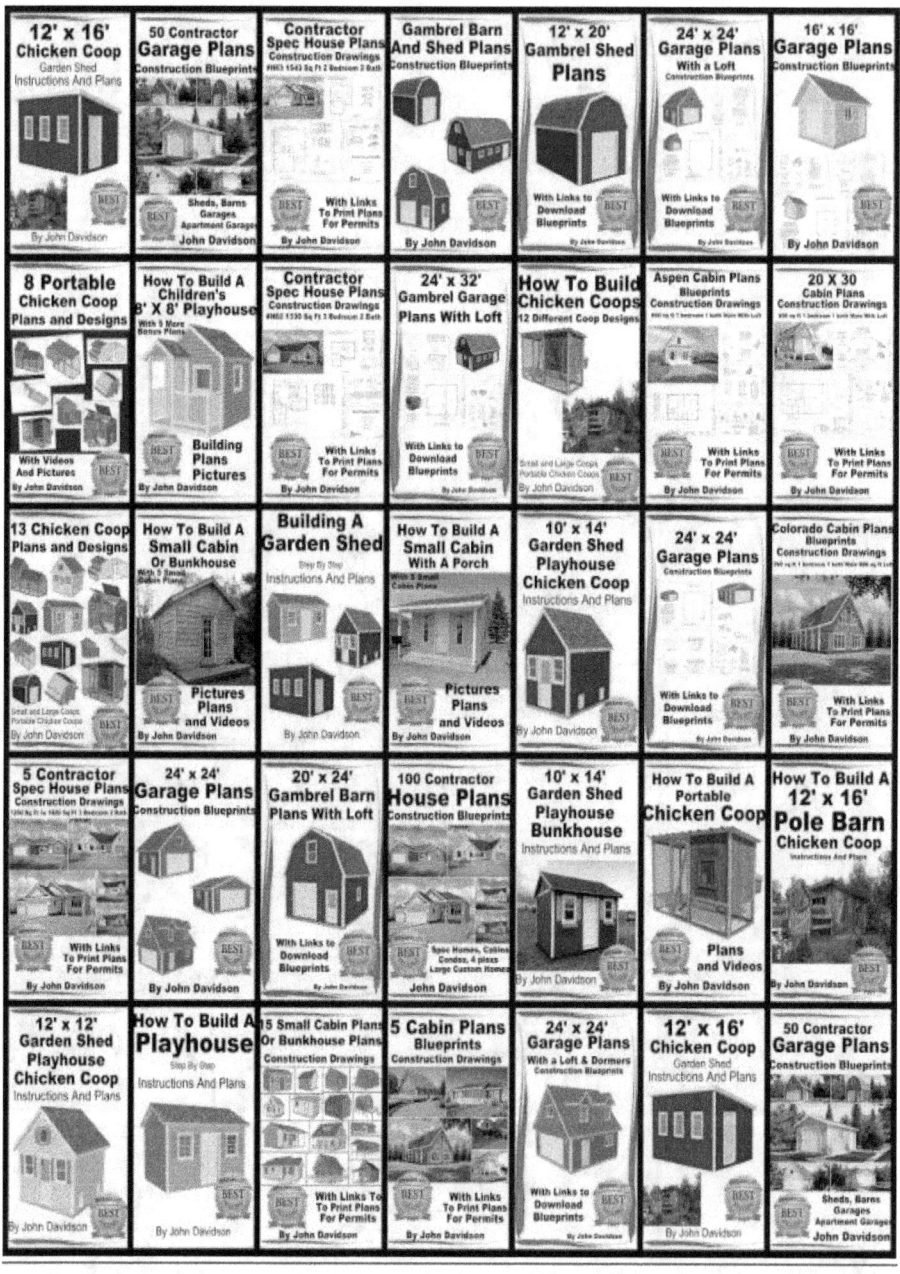

Entrepreneur Book Series

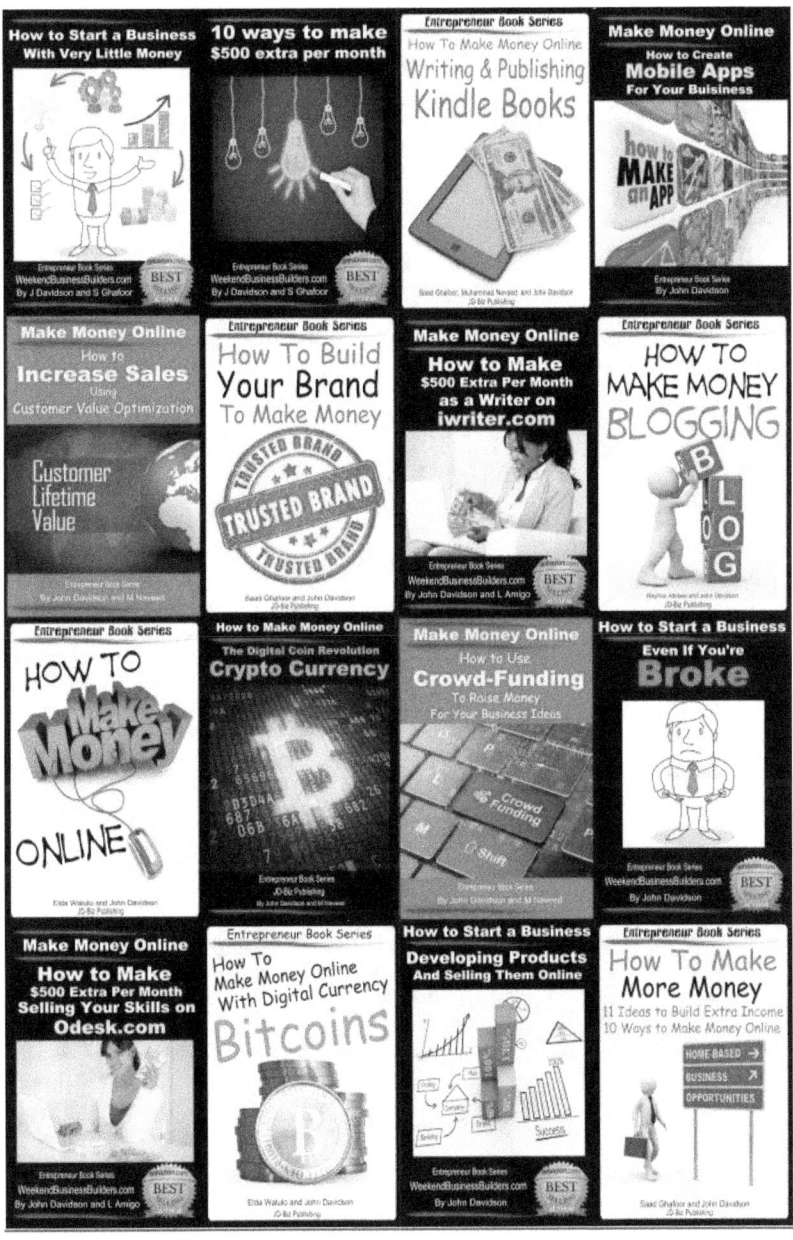

Our books are available at

1. Amazon.com

2. Barnes and Noble

3. Itunes

4. Kobo

5. Smashwords

6. Google Play Books

Publisher

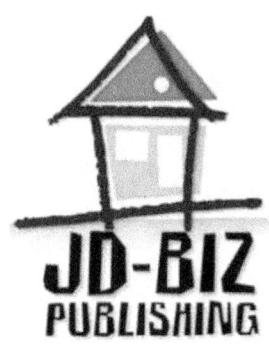

JD-Biz Corp

P O Box 374

Mendon, Utah 84325

http://www.jd-biz.com/

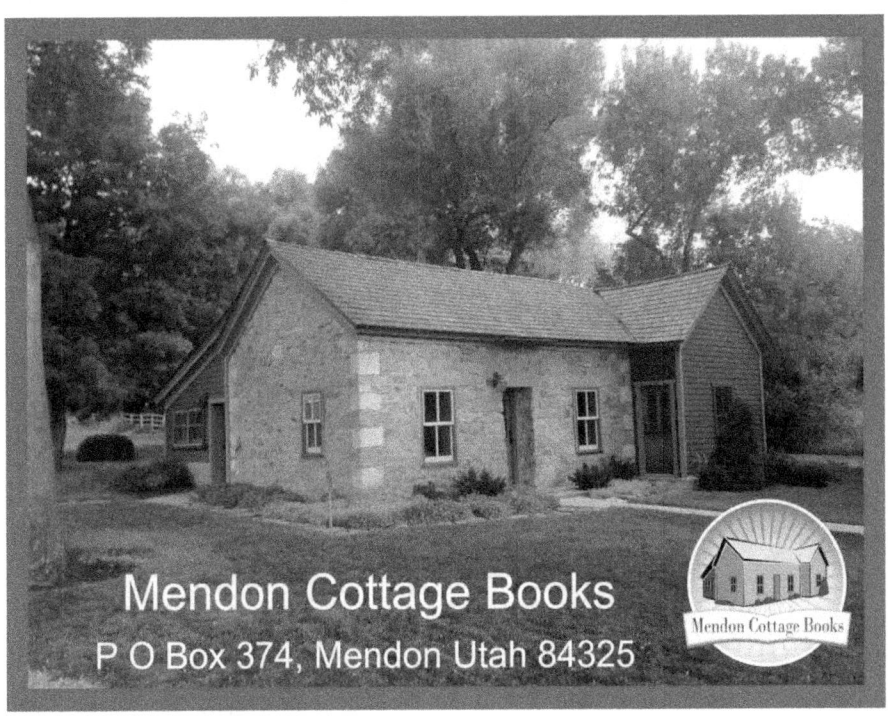

Mendon Cottage Books

P O Box 374, Mendon Utah 84325